20 Questions & Answers About Crohn's Disease

Francis A. Farraye, MD, MSc

Clinical Director, Section of Gastroenterology
Boston Medical Center
Professor of Medicine
Boston University School of Medicine
Boston, MA

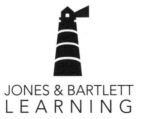

JONES & BARTLETT
LEARNING

World Headquarters

Jones & Bartlett Learning
5 Wall Street
Burlington, MA 01803
978-443-5000
info@jblearning.com
www.jblearning.com

Jones & Bartlett Learning
Canada
6339 Ormindale Way
Mississauga, Ontario L5V 1J2
Canada

Jones & Bartlett Learning
International
Barb House, Barb Mews
London W6 7PA
United Kingdom

The author, editor, and publisher have made every effort to provide accurate information. However, they are not responsible for errors, omissions, or for any outcomes related to the use of the contents of this book and take no responsibility for the use of the products and procedures described. Treatments and side effects described in this book may not be applicable to all people; likewise, some people may require a dose or experience a side effect that is not described herein. Drugs and medical devices are discussed that may have limited availability controlled by the Food and Drug Administration (FDA) for use only in a research study or clinical trial. Research, clinical practice, and government regulations often change the accepted standard in this field. When consideration is being given to use of any drug in the clinical setting, the healthcare provider or reader is responsible for determining FDA status of the drug, reading the package insert, and reviewing prescribing information for the most up-to-date recommendations on dose, precautions, and contraindications, and determining the appropriate usage for the product. This is especially important in the case of drugs that are new or seldom used.

Production Credits

Executive Publisher: Christopher Davis
Managing Editor for Custom Projects:
  Kathy Richardson
Associate Production Editor:
  Laura Almozara
Manufacturing and Inventory Control
  Supervisor: Amy Bacus
Composition: Spoke & Wheel

Cover Design: Kate Ternullo
Cover Images (from left): © Philip Date/
  ShutterStock, Inc.; © Monkey Business
  Images/ShutterStock, Inc.; © Olga
  Bogatyrenko/ShutterStock, Inc.
Printing and Binding: Malloy, Inc.
Cover Printing: Malloy, Inc.

ISBN-13: 978-1-4496-3731-6

6048

Printed in the United States of America
15 14 13 12 11 10 9 8 7 6 5 4 3 2 1

This book is written for my patients with inflammatory bowel disease.

It is dedicated to my loving and devoted family: my wife, Renee M. Remily, MD; my children, Jennifer and Alexis Farraye; and my parents, who taught me that hard work, perseverance, and commitment can result in great accomplishments.

I must acknowledge several individuals who made publication of this book possible. First, I thank Christopher Davis, Executive Publisher of Medicine at Jones & Bartlett Learning, for his confidence in my ability to bring this project to fruition. Also at Jones & Bartlett Learning, I would like to thank Special Projects Editor, Kathy Richardson, and Associate Production Editor, Laura Almozara.

I would like to thank my mentors and colleagues. With their encouragement, I developed skills as an inflammatory bowel disease expert and as a clinical investigator asking questions on ways to improve the lives of individuals with gastrointestinal disorders.

The Crohn's and Colitis Foundation is acknowledged for all the work they do for patients with inflammatory bowel disease and their efforts to cure Crohn's disease and ulcerative colitis, and to improve the quality of life of children and adults affected by these diseases. Finally, I thank my patients (and their families) for their confidence in allowing me to care for them. They are truly heroes.

CONTENTS

PART ONE

The Basics

What are the inflammatory bowel diseases?
What is Crohn's disease? Are there different
types of Crohn's disease?

What are the symptoms of Crohn's disease?

What is the difference between irritable bowel
syndrome and inflammatory bowel disease?

What causes Crohn's disease?

Inflammatory bowel disease (IBD)

A term for a variety of long-lasting disorders that cause inflammation in the gastrointestinal tract. The most common disorders are ulcerative colitis and Crohn's disease.

Small intestine

Organ where digestion and absorption occurs. It measures about 20 feet and includes the duodenum, jejunum, and ileum.

Ulcerative colitis

A disease that causes ulcers and irritation in the inner lining of the colon and rectum.

Crohn's disease

A form of inflammatory bowel disease that causes inflammation in the gastrointestinal (GI) tract. It usually affects the lower small intestine and/or the colon, but it can also affect any part of the GI tract. Also called regional enteritis, granulomatous colitis, and ileitis.

Chronic

Lasting for a long time.

1. What are the inflammatory bowel diseases? What is Crohn's disease? Are there different types of Crohn's disease?

The **inflammatory bowel diseases (IBD)** include diseases of the large and **small intestines**, such as **ulcerative colitis (UC)** and **Crohn's disease (CD)**. Inflammatory bowel disease is a **chronic** (long-lasting) disorder of unknown cause that results in inflammation of the **gastrointestinal (GI) tract**. While Crohn's disease can affect any part of the gastrointestinal (GI) tract, UC affects the **large intestine**, also called the **colon** (see **Figure 1**). There are other types of **inflammation** (irritation and swelling) in the colon, including **infectious colitis, ischemic colitis,** and **diverticulitis**. This book, however, focuses on questions about CD, which was first fully described in 1932, by Drs. Burrill Crohn, Leon Oppenheimer, and Gordon Ginzburg. They described Crohn's disease as inflammation of the **terminal ileum** (lower end of small intestine) and called the disease **regional enteritis** or **terminal ileitis**. CD can also affect the colon as well as the **perianal** (around the anus) area and upper gastrointestinal tract.

Crohn's disease most typically involves both the small intestine and colon, a condition called **ileocolitis**. However, CD is sometimes limited to either the small or large intestine. Isolated inflammation of the small intestine is called either **ileitis** or jejunioileitis, depending on the region of the small intestine that is affected. Isolated inflammation of the colon is called Crohn's colitis. The upper GI tract (stomach and **duodenum**) is involved approximately 5% of the time. Inflammation in Crohn's disease can be patchy, with areas of normal tissue surrounded by areas of inflammation (known as skip areas) (see **Figure 2**).

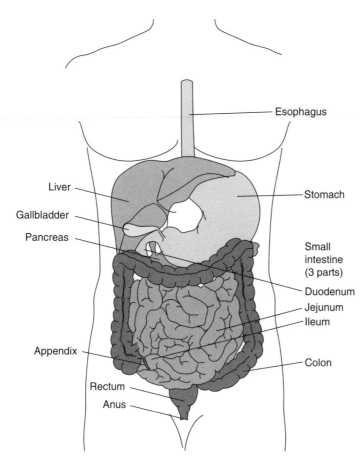

- Esophagus
- Liver
- Stomach
- Gallbladder
- Pancreas
- Small intestine (3 parts)
- Duodenum
- Jejunum
- Ileum
- Appendix
- Colon
- Rectum
- Anus

Figure 1 Normal gastrointestinal anatomy.

Another name for CD is **granulomatous colitis**; this is because under the microscope, **granulomas,** a collection of large inflammatory cells, are found in about 25% of patients with CD. Granulomas are not seen in patients with UC.

Although there are several layers that make up the intestines, the inflammation of UC involves only the innermost lining, called the colon **mucosa.** In contrast, CD can involve all the layers of the GI tract. As a result, there are complications unique to CD, including the development of a **fistula** and/or **abscess** (see Part 3 for additional information).

THE BASICS

Gastrointestinal (GI) tract

A large, muscular tube that extends from the mouth to the anus, where the movement of muscles, along with the release of hormones and enzymes, allows for the digestion of food. Also called the alimentary canal or digestive tract.

Large intestine

Part of the intestine that includes the appendix, cecum, colon, and rectum. The large intestine absorbs water from the stool and changes it from a liquid to a solid. The large intestine is four feet long.

Colon

Part of the large intestine extending from the cecum up to, but not including, the rectum.

Inflammation

Soreness, irritation, swelling.

Infectious colitis

Inflammation of the colon caused by a bacteria, parasite, or virus.

Ischemic colitis

Inflammation of the colon caused by decreased blood flow. It may cause bloody diarrhea.

Diverticulitis

A condition that occurs when small pouches in the colon, called diverticula, become inflamed.

Ileum

The lower end of the small intestine.

Terminal ileum

Distal 1–2 feet of the ileum. Attached to colon by the ileocecal valve.

Regional enteritis

Another name for Crohn's disease.

Terminal ileitis

Another name for Crohn's disease.

Perianal

The area around the anus.

ileocolitis

Inflammation of the lower part of the small intestine and the beginning part of the colon.

Ileitis

Inflammation of the small intestine. Several different disorders can cause inflammation of the small intestine.

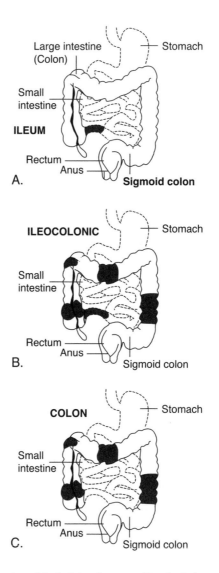

Figure 2 Location of Crohn's involvement. The shaded areas in figure **A** show terminal ileal involvement, while figure **B** shows involvement of the terminal ileum and colon, and figure **C** demonstrates isolated colonic involvement.

One recent study estimated the total direct cost of Crohn's disease in the United States at $3.1 billion per year. For Crohn's disease, 31% of costs were attributable to hospital costs, 33% to outpatient care, and 35%

to drug costs. The cost to society is even higher if you include the indirect costs for lost productivity.

Crohn's disease can present itself in a variety of ways. In some patients, chronic inflammation leads to narrowing of the intestines and development of a **stricture**, resulting in an intestinal blockage, while other individuals present with fistulae. Finally, the perianal area will be affected in as many as 30% of individuals with CD. The manifestations of perianal Crohn's disease include **fissures** (anal tears), **anal ulcers**, anal stenosis (narrowing of the anal canal), abscesses, and fistulae (see **Figure 3**).

There is no medical cure for CD, but most people can get effective treatment for their symptoms. Crohn's disease is a lifelong condition; there are medications that can be used to treat and manage CD (see Part 4). Some patients may benefit from surgery (see Part 6). Although there is no cure for CD, there are many ways to cope with the disease (see Part 8).

2. What are the symptoms of Crohn's disease?

The most common symptoms of CD are **abdominal** (stomach) discomfort; loose **stools** (bowel movements), which may contain blood and **mucus**; vomiting; fever; and weight loss. If the **rectum** (lower end of the large intestine) is involved, there may be significant **urgency** (the feeling of "needing to go"), in which the individual with CD needs to find a toilet quickly. Individuals with anal or perianal involvement may complain of anal discomfort, painful bowel movements, and rectal discharge; other symptoms include fatigue, fever, chills,

---

THE BASICS

Duodenum
The first part of the small intestine.

Granulomatous colitis
Another name for Crohn's disease of the colon.

Granuloma
Finding seen under the microscope in some patients with Crohn's disease.

Mucosa
The lining of the GI tract organs that absorbs nutrients and fluid, forms a barrier, and produces mucus.

There is no medical cure for CD, but most people can get effective treatment for their symptoms.

Fistula/Fistulae
An abnormal passage between two organs, or between an organ and the outside of the body, caused when inflamed tissues come into contact and join together.

Abscess

An accumulation of pus.

Sigmoid colon

Lower part of the colon that empties into the rectum.

Stricture

A narrowed area of intestine that develops due to chronic inflammation.

Fissure

A tear in the lining of the anal canal.

Anal ulcer

An ulcer within or just outside the anal canal.

Abdomen/ abdominal

Related to the area between the chest and the hips, consisting of the stomach, small intestine, large intestine, liver, gallbladder, pancreas, and spleen.

Stool

Solid waste that passes through the rectum as a bowel movement; it includes undigested food, bacteria, mucus, and dead cells. Also called feces.

Mucus

Clear to white liquid made by the intestines that coats and protects tissues in the gastrointestinal tract.

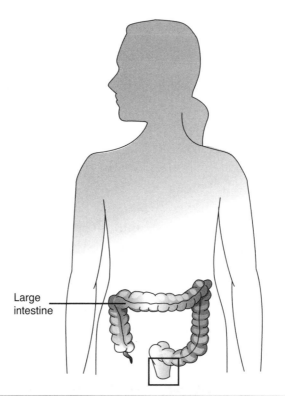

Large intestine

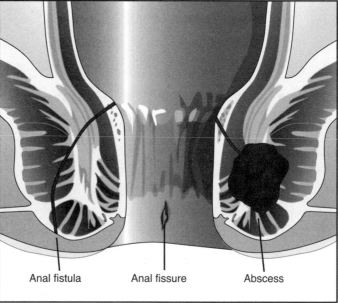

Anal fistula   Anal fissure   Abscess

Figure 3 Examples of an anal fistula, anal fissure, and perianal abscess.

and a loss of appetite. Symptoms vary between individuals. In addition to defining CD by the location, your **clinician** (doctor) may also define your CD as mild, moderate, or severe. The severity of CD is determined by a number of factors, including the frequency of loose stools or **diarrhea** and signs of toxicity (fever, rapid heart rate, and abnormal lab tests).

Some individuals have minimal symptoms, while others have more severe complaints. The severity of your symptoms is directly related to the extent of the inflammation in the small and large intestines. The more extensive the inflammation is, the worse the symptoms are. You can also have symptoms that involve the mouth, joints, skin, eyes, and liver. If CD develops during childhood or as a teenager, the affected individuals may not grow normally and may enter puberty later than other children their age. Symptoms of CD can come and go. When the CD symptoms are active, you are said to be having a **flare**. When the symptoms seem to go away for a while, you are in **remission**. In some individuals, it is possible to be in remission for years.

The symptoms of CD can be treated effectively in the majority of patients; however, there is no medical cure. Medications used to treat and manage CD are addressed in Part 4. As many as 75% of patients with CD may need surgery (Part 6).

Rectum

Lower end of the large intestine leading to the anus.

Urgency

The feeling of "needing to go" (either urine or stool).

Clinician

A healthcare professional engaged in the care of patients.

Diarrhea

Frequent, loose, and watery bowel movements. Causes include GI infections, irritable bowel syndrome, inflammatory bowel disease, medicines, and malabsorption.

Flare

Worsening of symptoms of disease.

Remission

Period of time when a disease does not cause symptoms.

THE BASICS

3. What is the difference between irritable bowel syndrome and inflammatory bowel disease?

Irritable bowel syndrome (IBS)

A disorder associated with abdominal pain, bloating, and altered bowel habits. Also called spastic colon or mucous colitis.

Although the names **irritable bowel syndrome (IBS)** and inflammatory bowel disease (IBD) sound alike, they are very different conditions. Irritable bowel syndrome is much more common than IBD. In fact, an estimated 15% of the US population has symptoms of IBS.

Patients with IBS have some similar symptoms as those with CD; these include diarrhea, abdominal cramps, and **bloating** (swelling of the abdomen). However, unlike CD, patients with IBS do not usually have weight loss, **rectal bleeding** (unless they also have bleeding hemorrhoids), fever, **anemia** (decreased red blood cell count), or symptoms that wake them at night. In addition, patients with IBS do not have the **extraintestinal** (outside the intestines) symptoms that can sometimes happen with CD, such as eye problems or mouth and skin ulcers. On the other hand, patients with IBS can develop a painful non-inflammatory joint and tissue condition called **fibromyalgia**.

Bloating

A fullness or swelling in the abdomen.

Rectal bleeding

Bleeding that comes out through the anus.

Anemia

Decreased red blood cells.

Extraintestinal

Occurring outside of the intestines.

Fibromyalgia

A chronic illness characterized by fatigue and widespread aching of muscles and soft tissues.

Overall, diagnosing and managing patients with CD can be difficult if they also have IBS. Crohn's disease affects men and women equally; IBS is nearly three times as common in women as it is in men. In particular, it may be more difficult to differentiate between CD and IBS based on symptoms alone. **Table 1** lists some of the similarities and differences between CD and IBS.

Table 1 Similarities and Differences Between Crohn's Disease and Irritable Bowel Syndrome

	CD	IBS
Symptoms in common	Diarrhea, abdominal cramps, and bloating	Diarrhea, abdominal cramps, and bloating
Different symptoms	Weight loss; rectal bleeding; fever; anemia; **nocturnal** symptoms; symptoms and findings related to the eyes, liver, skin, and joints	Not typically seen in IBS patients
Gender	Affects men and women equally	70% women, 30% men
Colonoscopy findings	Inflammation and/or ulcers	No visible inflammation
Pathology	Biopsies show inflammation with crypt abscesses, crypt branching	No inflammation seen
Treatments	5ASAs, corticosteroids, immuno-modulators, antibiotics, biologic agents, surgery	Diet, antispasmodics, tricyclics, lubiprostone, alosetron; no surgery
Pattern of illness	Periods of active disease (flare) and periods of remission	Symptoms can come and go

Nocturnal
Occurring at night.

4. What causes Crohn's disease?

Despite many theories, the causes for Crohn's disease remain unknown. CD is not contagious; you cannot "catch" it from a friend, family member, or acquaintance.

Although stress can cause changes in bowel habits, the inflammation characteristic of CD is not caused by stress. There is nothing you did or did not do that led to the development of CD.

There is nothing you did or did not do that led to the development of CD.

A combination of family (**genetic**) factors and exposure to something in the environment appear to be associated with the development of CD. Environmental factors

Genetic
Relating to biologic inheritance.

9

include intestinal infections, cigarette smoking, sanitation and hygiene, where you live in the world, and the use of certain medications. Although nonsteroidal anti-inflammatory drugs (NSAIDs), such as aspirin, ibuprofen, and naproxen, are used to reduce inflammation, in some studies, prolonged use of NSAIDs have been associated with flares of disease activity in patients with established CD. Low-dose aspirin (81 mg) is felt to be safe. Isotretinoin (formerly marketed as Accutane), a drug used to treat severe acne, has been associated in some studies with the development of IBD.

Although cigarette smoking may protect against the development of UC and limit symptoms, the opposite is true in individuals with CD. The risk of developing CD is two-fold higher in smokers compared to nonsmokers and the risk of developing recurrent CD after bowel resection is also higher in smokers. Nonetheless, it is strongly recommended that CD patients stop smoking.

The use of oral contraceptive pills and the development of IBD remain controversial. The most recent study suggests an association between the use of oral contraceptive agents and an increased risk of developing IBD, in particular CD. In this study, the risk of developing CD returns to normal after stopping the oral contraceptive agent. Be sure to consult with your doctor about the use of any medications, including oral contraceptives.

Cecum

The first part of the large intestine.

Appendectomy

Operation to remove the appendix.

Appendicitis

Inflammation of the appendix, typically causing severe pain in the lower right side of the abdomen.

The appendix is a 4-inch pouch attached to the **cecum**, the first part of the large intestine. Several studies have demonstrated that undergoing an **appendectomy** for confirmed **appendicitis** prior to the age of 20 is associated with a lower risk of developing ulcerative colitis. In contrast, some studies about Crohn's disease suggest an association between an appendectomy and an increased risk of developing Crohn's disease. However, many investigators believe that this association is artificial. They feel that the attack of appendicitis may have actually been the first presentation of Crohn's disease in which Crohn's symptoms are mistaken for appendicitis and an appendectomy done.

The degree to which the body's natural immunity is involved in the development of CD is not entirely understood. An abnormal **immune system** is felt to play a role in the development of CD. In patients with inflammatory bowel disease, there is an inappropriate response of the immune system in the lining of the intestine to normal bacteria and other proteins in the intestinal tract. An individual's genetic makeup may be a risk factor to this abnormal response. The fact that other body systems, such as the eyes and liver, are involved when CD is present favors a problem with the immune system. The current theory is that an individual inherits a predisposition to develop CD and then develops the disease after an exposure to an environmental trigger.

Immune system

A complex and intertwined system of cells and genetics that controls the body's defense system against infection and other foreign organisms or substances.

PART TWO

Risk Factors and Prevention

Who gets Crohn's disease?

Does Crohn's disease run in families?
Can I pass Crohn's disease to my children?

What factors can affect Crohn's disease?

5. Who gets Crohn's disease?

Both men and women can develop CD, and there are approximately 700,000 individuals in the United States living with the disease. The average age of onset of CD is between the ages of 15 and 35 years (25–30% of patients are diagnosed before the age of 20 years), but it can be diagnosed at any age. Approximately 30,000 new cases of ulcerative colitis and Crohn's disease are diagnosed yearly, and the rate of new cases of CD has been increasing since the 1940s. CD is not contagious; you cannot "catch" it from a friend, family member, or acquaintance.

Although anyone can get CD, there are certain groups of people for whom the risk is more likely. White individuals develop CD more commonly than other racial groups. Individuals of Jewish descent, especially of northern European origin, are 3 to 5 times more likely to be affected by IBD. Inflammatory bowel diseases are more common in the United States and Europe than in the developing countries of Africa and South America. However, even geographic areas where the incidence of IBD is low have seen increases in the number of new cases.

6. Does Crohn's disease run in families? Can I pass Crohn's disease to my children?

Yes, CD does run in families. As many as 1 in 5 individuals with CD have a family member who also has CD. The importance of genes in the development of CD is demonstrated by studies of identical twins. Research shows that if one identical twin has CD, then there is as high as a 60% chance that their twin will also develop CD. In addition to genetics, environmental exposures play an important role in the development of CD. Currently, there is no way to predict if a particular family member will develop CD; however, if you have CD, there is an increased chance that your children, brothers, and sisters will also develop the disease. Although there is no test presently available for a specific CD gene, the risk to your children has been estimated to be 8%, though higher rates have been reported in certain ethnic groups. Despite this increased risk, you should not dismiss the idea of having children.

7. What factors can affect Crohn's disease?

There are several things that can affect flare-ups in CD. For instance, **nonsteroidal anti-inflammatory drugs (NSAIDs)** are used by many people to treat aches and pain. Common NSAIDs include aspirin, naproxen, and ibuprofen. Some patients with UC can experience a flare of their colitis when taking NSAIDs. However, low-dose aspirin (81 mg) is felt to be safe. NSAIDs can sometimes cause upper abdominal discomfort and internal bleeding, in addition to other side effects. However, patients with CD can take acetaminophen safely. If you do need to take a NSAID, consider taking the lowest possible dose, take it with food, and take it for the shortest period of time possible. Additionally, some studies suggest that use of the acne drug isotretinoin may be associated with the development of IBD. Please talk to your doctor to determine what is best for you before taking any drugs.

Nonsteroidal anti-inflammatory drugs (NSAIDs)

A class of medications that can reduce pain, fever, and inflammation.

All patients with CD are strongly encouraged to stop smoking. Smoking in CD is associated with more flares, more complications, and an increased need for steroids and other medications, as well as an earlier recurrence of symptoms after surgery.

Fiber

A substance in foods that comes from plants. Fiber helps keep the stool soft so that it moves smoothly through the colon. Soluble fiber dissolves in water and is found in beans, fruit, and oat products. Insoluble fiber does not dissolve in water and is found in whole-grain products and vegetables.

Lactose intolerance

Being unable to digest lactose, the sugar in milk.

Celiac disease

An immune reaction to gluten, a protein found in wheat, rye, and barley. The disease causes damage to the lining of the small intestine and prevents absorption of nutrients. Also called celiac sprue, gluten intolerance, and nontropical sprue.

Gluten

A protein found in wheat, rye, and barley. In people with celiac disease, gluten damages the lining of the small intestine or causes sores on the skin.

Although many patients feel that their diet plays a role in their CD, there is no evidence to support that a specific diet can cause intestinal inflammation. However, when your CD is active or if you have a stricture, a low-**fiber** diet is suggested.

All individuals, regardless of CD, are encouraged to eat a well-balanced diet. If certain foods seem to increase diarrhea or abdominal pain, consider eliminating each food individually and see how your stomach reacts. Some individuals can have **lactose intolerance** (the inability to digest milk) in addition to CD. Finally, patients with IBD have an increased risk of **celiac disease** (an allergy to **gluten**), and should be tested for this disorder if symptoms are ongoing. A consultation with a nutritionist can be helpful.

As with diet, stress can cause many gastrointestinal symptoms, but there is no evidence to support that stress causes CD. If a patient feels stress in their life and is unable to cope with a CD diagnosis, their healthcare provider may have some helpful insight. See Question 17 about healthy coping and stress management.

PART THREE

Diagnosis

How does my doctor diagnose Crohn's disease?

How does my clinician know I don't
have ulcerative colitis?

What is a fistula? What is an abscess?

8. How does my doctor diagnose Crohn's disease?

Because loose stools (both bloody and non-bloody) can have other causes, your clinician will typically obtain stool samples to make sure there is no evidence of an infection that can mimic CD. Common bacteria that can cause infections leading to bloody diarrhea include *Salmonella*, *Shigella*, *Campylobacter*, and *E. coli* 0157. Rarely are bloody stools caused by a parasite or infection with *C. difficile*, a bacterium commonly associated with taking antibiotics and often acquired in hospitals. You don't need to travel to exotic places in the world to develop these infections: you can be exposed to them in nursing homes, hospitals, or restaurants. Stool samples are sent to a lab to determine if a bacterium is causing the diarrhea and examined to look for **ova** (the eggs of the parasites) and **parasites**.

Your healthcare provider may refer you to a **gastroenterologist** (a doctor who specializes in the digestive system) if your diarrhea continues and the stool samples fail to identify an infection. The gastroenterologist will take a detailed history and perform a physical examination. Examination of the perianal area may identify changes associated with anal Crohn's disease. He or she may ask about eye, skin, and joint symptoms, as these extraintestinal symptoms can be present in patients with CD. In some situations, joint pain, skin lesions, and eye symptoms may occur even before abdominal pain and diarrhea begin.

Blood tests will be done to look for inflammation, certain types of proteins associated with IBD, and anemia caused by blood loss. These tests include the following:

Ova

The eggs of the parasites.

Parasite

An infectious agent that lives in humans from which it obtains nutrition. Certain intestinal parasites can cause diarrhea and rectal bleeding.

Gastroenterologist

A doctor who specializes in the diagnosis and treatment of digestive diseases.

- CBC (complete blood count)
- Comprehensive **metabolic panel** (evaluates liver and kidney functions)
- ESR (erythrocyte sedimentation rate)
- Vitamin B12 and Vitamin D level
- CRP (C-reactive protein)

A complete blood count will be obtained to determine the white blood cell and red blood cell count, as the white blood cell count can be higher in patients with colitis. Similarly, chronic intestinal bleeding can cause a lower red blood cell count and the patient can develop anemia. A comprehensive metabolic panel evaluates your liver and kidney function to make sure these organs are working correctly. Blood tests for erythrocyte sedimentation rate (ESR) and C-reactive protein (CRP) are usually done to look for signs of inflammation. Vitamin B12 and Vitamin D are both absorbed in the small intestine and CD patients with small intestine problems can develop low levels of these vitamins. Vitamin B12 is important in the formation of blood cells and nervous system while Vitamin D is important for bone health. Vitamin D also plays a role in immunity. In some situations, blood might be tested to check for specific antibodies that are associated with CD.

Your gastroenterologist will then most likely perform a **sigmoidoscopy** or **colonoscopy** to examine the lining of your colon. A sigmoidoscopy is usually performed without **sedation** and uses a thin (about the size of your index finger), flexible tube with a light that is inserted into the rectum to examine the lower third of the colon. Preparation for a sigmoidoscopy requires the use of rectally administered **enemas** that empty the **lower bowel**.

Metabolic panel
Blood tests that measure several components including sodium, potassium, chloride, bicarbonate, blood urea nitrogen, creatinine, liver tests, calcium, and glucose.

Sigmoidoscopy
Looking into the sigmoid colon and rectum with a flexible tube called a sigmoidoscope.

Colonoscopy
A test to look into the rectum and colon that uses a long, flexible, narrow tube with a light and tiny camera on the end called a colonoscope.

Sedation
Administration of medications during a test to reduce anxiety and discomfort.

Enema
The insertion of a liquid medication into the rectum and lower colon as a treatment.

Lower bowel
Lower part of the colon that connects to the anus.

A picture of a normal ileum and an ileum affected by Crohn's disease, both taken at colonoscopy, are shown in **Figures 4** and **5**.

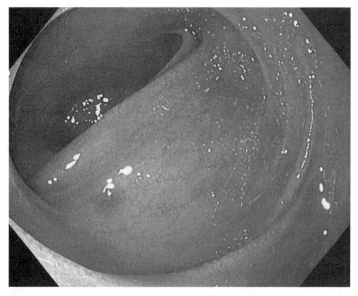

Figure 4 Normal small intestine as seen during colonoscopy.

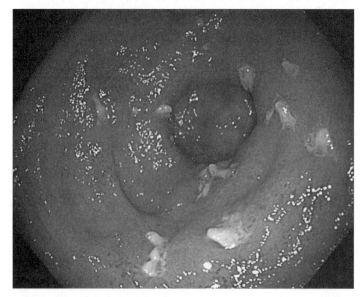

Figure 5 Ileum with ulcerations seen in a patient with Crohn's disease during colonoscopy.

You are unable to have any solid food the day before your colonoscopy. A laxative is given the night before the procedure to cleanse the bowel of stool, which allows your physician to get good views of the colon. More recently, clinicians have begun using a "split" dose of **bowel prep**, in which one dose is given the night before the procedure and one given early on the morning of your test. While you are lying on their left side, your gastroenterologist performs a rectal exam with a gloved and lubricated finger. The colonoscope (a long, flexible tube with a light and camera) is inserted into your anus up to the cecum and terminal ileum (see **Figure 6**).

Although flexible sigmoidoscopy is typically performed without sedation, sedation is given to nearly all patients undergoing colonoscopy. Mild cramping may be felt during the procedure, which can be reduced by taking several slow, deep breaths. Your gastroenterologist will also look for inflammation and abnormalities of the colon, such as **polyps** (growths) or **ulcers**. Tissue samples, called **biopsies**, are obtained during the procedure. The biopsied material is sent to a pathologist, who examines the tissue under a microscope. There are specific findings on the biopsy that can establish a diagnosis

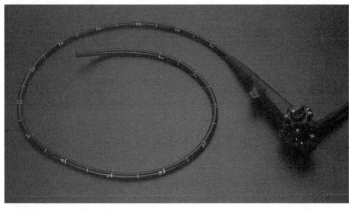

Figure 6 A colonoscope.

DIAGNOSIS

Bowel prep

Process used to clean the colon with enemas or a special drink that causes frequent bowel movements.

Polyp

An abnormal growth on the surface of the large or small intestine.

Ulcer

A sore on the skin's surface or on the stomach or intestinal lining.

Biopsy

A procedure in which a tiny piece of a body part, such as the colon, small intesine, or stomach, is removed for examination with a microscope.

of IBD. See **Figures 7** and **8,** which show a normal colon biopsy and one from a patient with CD. **Figure 9** is a microscopic image of a granuloma.

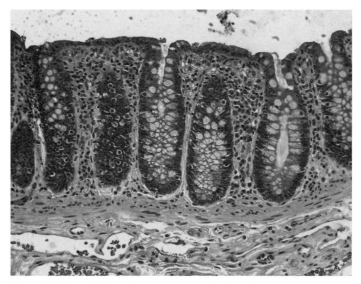

Figure 7 Normal colon tissue as seen under the microscope.

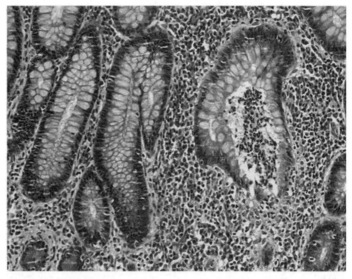

Figure 8 Inflammation characteristic of Crohn's disease as seen under the microscope.

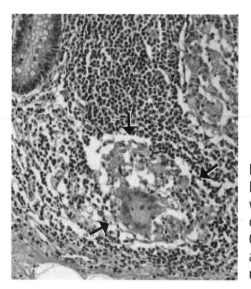

Figure 9
Inflammation with a granuloma characteristic of Crohn's disease as seen under the microscope.

It is important that a diagnosis of Crohn's disease be firmly established. Following your clinician's recommendations regarding testing will assist in proper diagnosis.

Depending on the symptoms, your clinician might also order X-rays of the small intestine, such as an **upper GI series** with a **small bowel X-ray** or a **CT scan** of the abdomen. Video capsule endoscopy is another method to evaluate the small intestine of individuals suspected of having CD. In this test, the individual swallows a pill-sized camera that takes more than 50,000 pictures over an 8-hour period, which are transmitted to a recording device that you wear. It is important that a diagnosis of Crohn's disease be firmly established. Following your clinician's recommendations regarding testing will assist in a proper diagnosis.

Upper GI series

X-rays of the esophagus, stomach, and duodenum. The patient swallows barium before X-rays are taken, as barium makes the organs show up on X-rays.

Small bowel X-ray

X-rays of the small intestine taken as barium liquid passes through the organ. Also called small bowel follow-through.

CT scan

An abbreviation for computed tomography, a technique of imaging body organs with detailed, cross-sectional views; it can be done with or without oral and intravenous contrast dye.

9. How does my clinician know I don't have ulcerative colitis?

Ulcerative colitis is the other major form of IBD. It also affects approximately 700,000 Americans, but unlike CD, which can affect the entire gastrointestinal tract (see Figure 9), UC only affects the rectum and colon, and in some situations the last few inches of the terminal ileum (**backwash ileitis**).

There are several layers that make up the colon, and ulcerative colitis and Crohn's disease involve different parts. The inflammation of UC involves only the innermost lining, called the mucosa (see **Figure 10**), but CD can affect all layers of the gastrointestinal tract.

There are features found on colonoscopy and biopsy that can help gastroenterologists distinguish CD from UC. While UC always involves the rectum, the rectum is affected in only 10–20% of individuals with CD. Inflammation of the rectum is called **proctitis**. X-rays of the

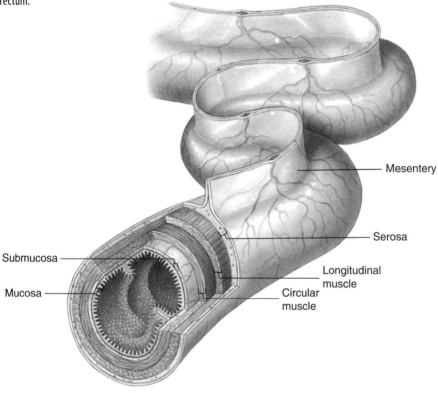

Figure 10 Cross-section of the layers of the small intestine.

abdomen can also help distinguish CD from UC. **MRI scans**, which use magnetic field energy to make images of your organs, are being performed more frequently as an alternative to CT scans, as there is no radiation exposure during a MRI. Although CD can involve the stomach and small intestines, UC does not. As noted in Part 1, granulomas are found under the microscope in about 25% of patients with CD, but these are not seen in patients with UC. Rectal bleeding is less common in patients with CD. Carefully listening to and analyzing symptoms, performing a physical exam, and using a combination of tests typically enables the clinician to distinguish CD from UC. In about 10% of cases, it may be difficult to distinguish CD from UC of the colon; this is called **indeterminate colitis**.

Table 2 shows a list of features that can be helpful in distinguishing CD from UC. There are also differences in the tissue biopsied from the affected part of the GI tract; see **Table 3** for an explanation of these differences.

MRI scan

A magnetic resonance imaging (MRI) scan is a test that uses a magnetic field and pulses of radio wave energy to make pictures of organs and structures inside the body.

Indeterminate colitis

Inflammation of the colon that cannot be easily classified as either ulcerative colitis or Crohn's disease.

10. What is a fistula? What is an abscess?

Because the ulcers from Crohn's disease can penetrate the entire wall of the intestine, a fistula and/or abscess can develop (see **Figure 3**, page 6). Fistulas are abnormal connections between two adjacent organs. Fistulas can be between organs, such as the bladder and bowel (enterovesical), rectum and vagina (rectovaginal), or the bowel and adjacent loop of bowel (enteroenteric). External fistulas can develop between the intestine and the skin (enterocutaneous). Fistulas develop in between 20 and 40% of patients with CD. In as many as 50% of patients, the fistula can develop prior to the diagnosis of CD. Symptomatic fistulae can be treated with medications (Part 4) and surgery (Part 6).

Table 2 Clinical Differences Between Ulcerative Colitis and
Crohn's Disease

Clinical Characteristic	Ulcerative Colitis	Crohn's Disease
Diarrhea	Typical	Typical
Rectal bleeding	Typical	Occurs
Abdominal mass	Not seen	Occurs
Mucosal disease	Continuous from rectum	Patchy (skip lesions)
Pseudopolyps	Seen	Seen
Rectal involvement	Characteristic	Occurs
Fistula	Not seen	Occurs
Perianal disease	Not seen	Occurs
Toxic megacolon	Occurs	Rare
Small bowel involvement	Not seen	Common
Cancer	Occurs (colon)	Occurs
pANCA blood test	60–70%	15%
pASCA blood test	15%	65%

pANCA

Anti-neutrophil cytoplasmic antibody blood test detected in autoimmune disorders.

pASCA

Anti-saccharomyces cerevisiae antibody blood test detected in autoimmune disorders.

An abscess, a collection of pus, can occur within the abdomen or around the anal area. A fistula can lead to the development of an abscess. Small abscesses can be treated with antibiotics, while larger abscesses are generally drained by inserting a needle into the abscess, which allows the pus to escape.

Table 3 Pathologic Differences between Ulcerative Colitis and Crohn's Disease

Clinical Characteristic	Ulcerative Colitis	Crohn's Disease
Depth	Mucosal	Transmural (full thickness of the colon or small intestine)
Crypt abscesses	Seen	Seen
Architecture distortion	Seen	Seen
Granuloma	Not seen	Occurs
Mesenteric fat, nodes	Not involved	Involved

PART FOUR

Treatment Options

What are the different types of medications
used to treat Crohn's disease?

If I am feeling well, why do I have
to keep taking my medications?

5-ASAs

Aminosalicylates are medications used to treat the inflammation associated with inflammatory bowel disease; they come in oral and topical forms.

Immunomodulators

A type of drug that is capable of modifying (decreasing or weakening) the effectiveness of the immune system.

Corticosteroid

A type of medication given to reduce inflammation. Corticosteroids come in oral and topical forms.

Biologic agents

A group of therapeutic medications that include monoclonal antibodies.

Retention enema

Insertion of medicated fluids through the anus into the rectum and lower colon to help heal inflammation.

Suppositories

A small plug of medication inserted in the rectum.

Intravenous (IV)

Given into a vein.

Tumor necrosis factor (TNF)

A type of protein that promotes inflammation in the body and gastrointestinal tract.

11. What are the different types of medications used to treat Crohn's disease?

Several types of medications are used to treat patients with CD. The major types include the **5-ASAs, immunomodulators, corticosteroids**, antibiotics and **biologic agents**.

The 5-ASA (aminosalicylates) agents are usually taken by mouth and act to reduce inflammation, but they do not affect the immune system. In addition to oral preparations, other 5-ASA treatments include **retention enemas** and **suppositories**.

Immunomodulators are used in patients who do not respond to anti-inflammatory medications (5-ASAs). Although these medications reduce the inflammation of CD, they (among other things) can also decrease the body's immune system function and increase the risk of infections. Patients on immunomodulators need regular monitoring of their blood to look for decreased red and white blood cells, as well as elevation in the liver function tests (which are possible side effects of the medications).

Like immunomodulators, corticosteroids also act on the immune system and are used in oral, rectal, and **intravenous (IV)** forms. Corticosteroids reduce the inflammation associated with CD and are in a class of drugs called anti-inflammatories. Although very effective for short-term use, there is a long list of side effects in patients chronically treated with corticosteroids.

Biologic agents are drugs that target specific proteins in the body. Some biologic agents block the production of **tumor necrosis factor (TNF)**. TNF is a protein that circulates in the blood and is associated with inflammation in the intestines. Another class of biologic agents targets the **adhesion molecules** that allow white blood cells to stick to the wall of the intestines.

Antibiotics are used to treat colonic CD, as well as infectious complications of abscesses. They are also used to treat perianal fistulae in individuals with CD and infections that may result from being on immunomodulators or corticosteroids.

A liquid diet of predigested nutrients, called an **elemental diet**, has been successfully used to treat children with CD. In this case, no regular food is allowed, with all nutrition derived from the elemental diet. As most individuals think that an elemental diet tastes bad, placement of a **nasogastric (NG) tube** is required to administer the liquid diet. Newer formulations taste better and may not require an NG tube.

Many individuals are using **prebiotics** and **probiotics** to treat IBD. Prebiotics are nondigestible nutrients that help promote the growth of "good" bacteria in your body. Probiotics are the actual "good" bacteria themselves in the form of a dietary supplement. Data supporting the use of prebiotics and probiotics is limited.

In some situations, agents that help reduce the spasms of pain and the bouts of diarrhea are used in combination with the above medications to treat the symptoms of abdominal cramps and frequent loose stools.

Acetaminophen is the preferred pain medication for use in patients with IBD. You should not use narcotic medications chronically, given the potential for addiction. Patients with chronic pain unrelated to active colitis might benefit from a referral to a comprehensive pain center.

Adhesion molecules

Proteins that help white blood cells stick to the lining of the intestines.

Elemental diet

A liquid diet of predigested nutrients used to treat patients with Crohn's disease.

Nasogastric (NG) tube

A tube inserted through the nose, down the esophagus, and into the stomach.

Prebiotics

Nondigestible food ingredients that are ingested by the normal bacteria occurring in the colon. They are believed to aid in digestion.

Probiotics

Live beneficial bacteria found in food or diet supplements; they are believed to aid in digestion and may decrease gastrointestinal symptoms.

TREATMENT OPTIONS

Crohn's disease can recur after surgery, so medications may be started soon after surgery in individuals at high risk for recurrent CD in an effort to decrease the chance that the CD will return. Close follow-up with a gastroenterologist is important after surgery.

12. If I am feeling well, why do I have to keep taking my medications?

It is not surprising that many healthcare providers feel that patients should stay on their medications even when they are feeling well.

Many patients with chronic disorders stop taking their medications or miss doses, and studies show that 43–72% of patients with IBD do not take their medications as prescribed.

Statistics show that those who stop their medication are more likely to be male, single, have limited inflammation, and taking rectally administered or multiple medications. Several research studies have demonstrated that patients with UC who do not take their medications are five times more likely to develop a flare of their colitis.

Relapse

Disease symptoms that recur after being in remission.

Colorectal cancer

Cancer that starts in the colon (also called the large intestine) or the rectum (the end of the large intestine).

Aside from the discomfort of a flare-up, evidence suggests that severe colon inflammation seen on colonoscopy and/or on colon biopsies may increase risk of colitis **relapse**, need for surgery to remove the colon, or development of **colorectal cancer**. Because several of the commonly used CD medications work to heal the inner lining of the colon, it is not surprising that many healthcare providers feel that patients should stay on their medications even when they are feeling well. Please talk with your healthcare provider before discontinuing any medication, to discuss the risks and benefits. There may be ways to change the medication routine to make it more convenient.

PART FIVE

Complications

What is my risk of developing colon cancer?
Is there anything I can do to decrease my risk?
How is chromoendoscopy used to diagnose
colon cancer?

13. What is my risk of developing colon cancer? Is there anything I can do to decrease my risk? How is chromoendoscopy used to diagnose colon cancer?

Colorectal cancer (CRC), which includes cancer of the colon and rectum, is one of the most feared complications of CD for patients and physicians alike. More than 135,000 cases of CRC are diagnosed annually in the United States, making it the second most common cancer. Patients with UC or Crohn's disease comprise 1–2% of new CRC cases.

It is important to note that the overwhelming majority of patients with CD will *not* develop colon cancer. In fact, recent studies suggest that the risk of developing colon cancer is significantly lower than previously thought.

Colonic CD

Crohn's disease isolated to the large intestine (colon and rectum).

Patients with certain types of CD are at increased risk of developing colon cancer, with the highest risk group including patients with extensive **colonic CD**. Patients with long-standing and extensive small intestinal Crohn's disease are also at an increased risk of developing small intestinal cancer. Patients with limited Crohn's disease of the colon are not at any higher risk than the general population.

The risk of developing CRC increases after approximately 8 years of being affected by Crohn's disease. This timeline is based on the onset of symptoms, not on the time when the diagnosis was made by a healthcare provider. The following are the factors for you and your clinician to consider when assessing risk for CRC:

- Extent of colonic inflammation
- Severity of colonic inflammation

- Duration of CD from onset of symptoms
- Family history of colon cancer in **first-degree relatives** (parents, siblings, or children)
- A first-degree relative diagnosed with CRC younger than 50 years of age
- Presence of **primary sclerosing cholangitis** (inflammation of the bile ducts)

At this time, it is not clear if children diagnosed with CD are at an increased risk of developing CRC (compared to adults), given that children have CD for a longer time. It is suggested that children, like adults, should follow screening recommendations.

All patients should undergo a colonoscopy 8–10 years after the onset of symptoms of colitis. Biopsies will be taken throughout the colon. At that time, the extent of the disease can be determined by the results of the biopsies and visual appearance of the lining of the colon. Typically, patients with more extensive colitis undergo a colonoscopy every 1–3 years after their initial screening colonoscopy and then every 8–10 years after the onset of symptoms. The interval between colonoscopies depends on the number of the risk factors described above; however, patients with primary sclerosing cholangitis should have a colonoscopy every year after the diagnosis is made.

The good news is that the risk of developing colorectal cancer for patients with Crohn's disease is decreasing. The lower risk may be related to widespread use of effective medical therapy, more frequent colonoscopies, and the use of **colectomy** (the surgical removal of all or part of the colon) in selected patients. Some individuals at higher risk for CRC may benefit from being in a surveillance program that includes regular colonoscopies.

COMPLICATIONS

First-degree relative

Mother, father, sister, brother, son, or daughter.

Primary sclerosing cholangitis (PSC)

Irritation, scarring, and narrowing of the bile ducts inside and outside the liver. Bile builds up in the liver, damaging its cells and in some cases leading to cirrhosis. Many people with this condition also have inflammatory bowel disease.

The good news is that the risk of developing colorectal cancer for patients with Crohn's disease is decreasing.

Colectomy

A surgical procedure to remove all or part of the colon.

To decrease the risk of developing CRC, here are some things that you can do:

- Be aware of risk factors
- Consult with a healthcare provider about remaining on medications to prevent relapses (a return of symptoms) and control inflammation in the colon
- Comply with the schedule of colonoscopies as developed by a clinician

Chromoendoscopy

A procedure in which dye is sprayed on the lining of the colon to make it easier to identify abnormalities during a colonoscopy.

Chromoendoscopy is a technique used to detect abnormalities in the colon of patients with CD. As discussed previously, patients with extensive and long-standing CD have an increased risk of developing colorectal cancer. Presently, multiple random biopsies of the colon are obtained during colonoscopy to screen for CRC. Any suspicious abnormalities observed by the gastroenterologist are also biopsied during the colonoscopy.

Chromoendoscopy entails spraying the colon with a dye that stains the lining and allows your doctor to identify more easily suspicious areas and biopsy them. The staining is not permanent and has no lasting effect on your colon. The two stains most commonly used are indigo carmine and methylene blue. Several studies have demonstrated that the colonoscopy and chromoendoscopy together can identify more serious abnormalities than random biopsies, but colonoscopy with chromoendoscopy may take more time than standard colonoscopy. At present, chromoendoscopy is reserved for patients at an increased risk of developing cancer or for those patients in whom suspicious findings were identified on earlier procedures.

PART SIX

Surgery

How often is surgery needed in patients with Crohn's disease and what operations are typically performed? What are the potential complications of surgery for Crohn's disease?

How is perianal Crohn's disease treated surgically?

14. How often is surgery needed in patients with Crohn's disease and what operations are typically performed? What are the potential complications of surgery for Crohn's disease?

Up to 75% of patients with Crohn's disease will require surgery. Surgery is not curative for Crohn's disease, but rather performed for several reasons, including:

- Intestinal obstruction (blockage)
- **Perforation** (bursting of the small or large intestine)
- Failure of medical therapy to relieve symptoms and induce remission
- **Dysplasia** (precancerous changes detected during colonoscopy) or colorectal cancer
- Side effects of treatment become severe or life-threatening
- Perianal disease
- **Toxic megacolon** (dilation of the colon that can occur in the setting of a severe attack of CD)
- Anemia (low red blood cell count related to bleeding and decreased red cell production by the bone marrow cells)

Several different types of operations are typically performed in patients with Crohn's disease. In patients with a stricture, the surgeon will remove the diseased segment of the intestines and attach the two normal ends together. The point of the new connection is called an **anastomosis**. Different types of anastomoses include connecting the small bowel to another segment of the small bowel, the small bowel to the colon (ileocolonic anastomosis) or the colon to another segment of colon

Perforation

The breaking open of an organ.

Dysplasia

A precancerous change in the lining of the gastrointestinal tract.

Toxic megacolon

Life-threatening complication usually from IBD that results in dilatation of the colon and possible perforation; may require emergency surgery to remove the colon.

Anastomosis/ Anastomoses

A surgically-created connection of two normally separate organs.

(colo-colonic anastomosis). Another approach is to try to open and repair the stricture without removing the segment of small intestines; this procedure is called a **stricturoplasty**. A stricturoplasty has been found to work well in individuals with short areas of small intestinal scarring without associated inflammation and is performed to conserve intestines.

In some patients with extensive rectal and colonic disease, the entire colon is removed (total proctocolectomy) and an **ostomy** is performed. An **ileostomy** (**Figure 11**) is when the surgeon makes an incision into the abdominal wall near the belt line and a loop of small intestine is brought through the opening and attached to the skin.

Stricturoplasty

An operation performed in patients with Crohn's disease to relieve obstruction of the small intestine without removal of the affected intestines.

Ostomy

An operation that makes it possible for stool to leave the body through an opening made in the abdomen. An ostomy is necessary when part or all of the intestines are removed or blocked. Colostomy and ileostomy are types of ostomies.

Ileostomy

An operation that attaches the small intestine to an opening in the abdomen called a stoma. An ostomy pouch, attached to the stoma and worn outside the body, collects stool.

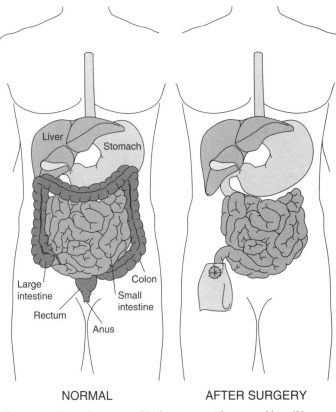

NORMAL

AFTER SURGERY

Figure 11 Normal anatomy (L); Ileostomy with external bag (R).

A bag is worn by the patient and emptied of stool several times a day. If a limited colon resection is performed, a **colostomy** is placed. A colostomy and ileostomy are similar, but in a colostomy a loop of colon is attached to the abdominal wall.

Laparoscopic bowel resections are being performed more commonly over the past several years. The surgeon makes several small incisions into your abdomen and inserts a sterile scope with a camera at the tip through the incision to access and remove the diseased intestines. This approach results in smaller scars and typically is associated with shorter hospital stays.

It is very beneficial to be in good physical condition prior to surgery. In some situations, nutrition is given through a vein to malnourished individuals before elective surgery.

Crohn's disease can come back after surgery, and you may require additional operations. It is important that you follow up with your gastroenterologist soon after surgery. In some cases treatment is started immediately after the surgery in an effort to decrease the chance of the Crohn's disease coming back. If multiple operations are performed on the small intestines and long segments of bowel are removed, there is a risk of **short bowel syndrome**. Individuals with short bowel syndrome are unable to absorb the food that they eat, resulting in diarrhea, nutrient deficiencies, and weight loss.

Patients often delay surgery, but keep in mind that appropriately timed surgery can lead to a dramatic improvement in your quality of life. Most patients are

Colostomy

An operation that attaches the colon to an opening in the abdomen called a stoma. An ostomy pouch, attached to the stoma and worn outside the body, collects stool.

Patients often delay surgery, but it is important to remember that appropriately timed surgery can lead to a dramatic improvement in your quality of life.

Short bowel syndrome

Problems related to absorbing nutrients after removal of a long segment of the small intestine. Symptoms include diarrhea, weakness, and weight loss.

happy with their decision to have surgery. However, as with many types of surgery, there can be short- and long-term complications. Some possible short-term complications include wound infection and abscesses, both of which can be treated with antibiotics. If there are non-healing leaks around the anastomoses or abscesses that do not respond to antibiotics, further surgery may be necessary.

Long-term complications may include **bowel obstruction** (blockage) from adhesions or recurrent CD. Bowel obstruction that does not respond to more conservative measures, like placement of a nasogastric tube, may require further surgery.

15. How is perianal Crohn's disease treated surgically?

Individuals with Crohn's disease can develop **anal fissures** (small tears in the anus), anal ulcers, perianal abscesses, and fistulae. You might complain of anal pain and rectal discharge. A MRI scan is often performed to define the location of the fistula and exclude an abscess. In most cases, the surgeon will then perform an examination under anesthesia to confirm the diagnosis and treat any local abscesses. In uncomplicated cases, a procedure called a **fistulotomy** is performed that can heal the fistula. To help relieve pain and speed healing, taking frequent warm baths called **sitz baths** may also be recommended. In other cases, the surgeon can place drains to keep abscesses from re-forming. Typically, a **seton** is placed in the track of the fistula to keep it open while medical treatment is started.

Bowel obstruction

A partial or complete blockage of the small or large intestine.

Anal fissure

A small tear in the anus that may cause itching, pain, or bleeding

Fistulotomy

An operation performed by a surgeon to treat an anal fistula.

Sitz bath

A special plastic tub that allows a person to sit in a few inches of warm water to help relieve the discomfort of hemorrhoids or anal fissures.

Suture

Material used during surgery to attach two structures.

Seton

A **suture**, made of thread or flexible wire, that is passed through a fistula to keep it open and prevent abscess formation.

PART SEVEN

Crohn's Disease in Older Adults

Can Crohn's disease develop
much later in life?

16. Can Crohn's disease develop much later in life?

Although most individuals with CD are diagnosed between the ages of 15 and 35 years, about 15% of new cases of IBD are diagnosed in individuals over the age of 65 years. At this age, there are a number of other conditions a physician may test for that can present with similar symptoms of CD. Some of these disorders include ischemic colitis, colon cancer, and diverticulosis.

Ischemic colitis occurs when blood flow is reduced to part of the colon, causing severe pain and bleeding. **Diverticulosis** is a common condition in which tiny pouches of tissue, called **diverticula**, poke through weak areas in the colon. Patients with diverticulosis can develop severe rectal bleeding. If the diverticula become infected, the condition is called diverticulitis, which causes abdominal pain and fever.

Although treating CD in older adults is basically the same as in younger patients, there are some differences:

- Older, frail patients may have difficulty administering and retaining enema therapy
- There may be a slower response to medical therapy in older adults
- Due to an increased number of preexisting conditions in older adults, they are at an increased risk for complications and interactions with other drugs they may be taking
- Elderly patients appear to have an increased risk of infectious complications when on steroids, immunomodulators, and biologic agents

Diverticulosis

A common condition in which tiny pouches of tissue, called diverticula, poke through weak areas of the colon.

Diverticula

Plural for diverticulum, a small outpouching in the colon. These pouches are not painful and can become inflamed and lead to rectal bleeding.

PART EIGHT

Coping and Surviving

Does stress cause Crohn's disease? Can stress affect my symptoms?

I am sick and have trouble making it to work every day. How can I work with my employer to help them understand my health situation?

17. Does stress cause Crohn's disease? Can stress affect my symptoms?

Doctors used to think that inflammatory bowel disease was caused by excessive stress. Today, scientific studies have shown no increase in the risk of developing the first symptoms of IBD after major life stress (such as the loss of a job or the death of a loved one). Studies also suggest that individuals under excessive stress do not develop CD more than others.

Many patients are convinced that their CD becomes active during stressful times in their lives. There is no question that active symptoms of Crohn's disease can create stress and, when stressed, you can develop abdominal cramps and a tendency towards looser stools. It is important to learn the difference between abdominal pain and diarrhea caused by stress and when it is a flare-up of CD. Having diarrhea and abdominal pain does not always mean that the inflammation in your intestines has worsened. It's still not clear if stress causes intestinal inflammation to become worse, but regardless of the cause, efforts to reduce stress can be very helpful.

Some researchers feel that perceived stress (that is, the way that you view your own stress) is more consistently linked to an increase in symptoms of IBD. In some studies, chronic perceived stress could predict future IBD relapses, suggesting there may be a buildup of the damaging effects of stress over time.

Treatments such as **relaxation therapies, psychotherapy**, and **cognitive-behavioral therapy** have been tried with IBD patients. These therapies sometimes improve well-being, provide coping strategies for the disease, and reduce psychological distress, but there is as yet

Relaxation therapies

Techniques such as deep breathing or imagery that allow a person to relax and relieve anxiety.

Psychotherapy

Treatment of emotional problems by a therapist using a variety of communication techniques.

Cognitive-behavioral therapy

A therapeutic approach that helps individuals take control of the way they respond to illness.

no objective evidence that they improve the underlying inflammation.

You are encouraged to speak to your clinician about how CD is affecting your daily activities. Active disease is stressful, and psychological therapies can be helpful in coping more effectively with the distress of the disease. Some gastroenterology offices have a relationship with a psychologist or psychiatrist who has experience with patients who have CD. Patients may also consider participating in stress reduction techniques like meditation and yoga. The Crohn's and Colitis Foundation of America (CCFA) sponsors support groups throughout the country. Many individuals find comfort in speaking to others with the same condition. See the CCFA Web site (http://www.ccfa.org) for a listing of support groups in your community.

It is not uncommon for Crohn's disease patients to fear attacks of pain and diarrhea and be tempted to stay close to home. However, there are some things you can do to prepare if symptoms should develop:

- Plan ahead: know the location of public restrooms. In some states, the Restroom Access Law allows access to all bathrooms in retail establishments for those having a note from their healthcare provider stating they have CD.

- If traveling on public transportation, try to sit as close to a restroom as possible.

- Carry some toilet paper, flushable wipes, and an extra set of underwear. Some people with CD may wear pads or disposable undergarments.

- Patients should consult with their clinician about taking anti-diarrheal medications at the first sign of cramping if they are not near a restroom.

When traveling further away, patients should consult with their clinician to make sure they have enough medication. Carrying a copy of key medical records, like a colonoscopy or CT scan report, is recommended. They should also ask for a list of gastroenterologists who practice in the area where they are visiting.

As stress is unavoidable today, you shouldn't hesitate to speak with your healthcare provider about methods to help improve your coping skills.

As stress is unavoidable today, patients shouldn't hesitate to speak with their healthcare provider about methods to help improve their coping skills. Finally, it is important that they understand that no matter how stressed they were before they developed colitis, the stress did not cause it.

18. I am sick and have trouble making it to work every day. How can I work with my employer to help them understand my health situation?

Patients who have a chronic illness like IBD may be covered under the Americans with Disabilities Act (ADA). They may also be eligible for time off under the Family and Medical Leave Act (FMLA). The ADA has been in effect since 1992 and prohibits private employers, state and local governments, employment agencies, and labor unions from discriminating against qualified individuals with disabilities. Under the ADA, employers are required to make a reasonable accommodation to those with a known disability if it would not impose an undue hardship on the operation of the employer's business.

To be protected by the ADA, one must have a disability, which is defined as a physical or mental impairment that substantially limits one or more major life activities;

a history or record of such impairment; or be perceived by others as having such impairment. An important amendment went into effect on January 1, 2009, that has a major impact on individuals with IBD. In this amendment, abnormalities in gastrointestinal functions are specifically included and are covered as a disability.

You can visit the CCFA Web site (http://www.ccfa.org/living/disability/) for more information. Examples of reasonable accommodations might include:

- Allowing enough time for frequent restroom breaks
- Moving an employee's workstation closer to a restroom
- Time off or unpaid leave for doctor's appointments, flare-ups, or hospitalizations
- Providing flexible work schedules or telecommuting opportunities
- Reassignment to a different position

The Family and Medical Leave Act, passed in 1993, provides eligible employees with a total of up to 12 work weeks of leave during a 12-month period for a variety of reasons, including taking medical leave when the employee is unable to work because of a serious health condition. The FMLA applies to all public agencies (state, local, and federal), including schools, and to private-sector businesses that employ 50 or more employees. To be eligible, you must have been working for the same employer for at least 12 months, putting in at least 1,250 hours during the previous 12 months, and at a location where at least 50 employees live within 75 miles of the worksite.

If a patient is having difficulty with their employer, they should ask their healthcare provider to write a letter describing their condition, treatment plans, and

Prognosis

Prediction of the course of disease.

prognosis. Contact a local Crohn's and Colitis Foundation of America (CCFA) chapter or call their toll free number (800-932-2423) to see if they are aware of local resources, including local government agencies or attorneys, who are able to assist in obtaining coverage under the ADA or FMLA laws.

PART NINE

Miscellaneous Issues and Resources

Should I get a second opinion?

Where can I get more information
about Crohn's disease?

19. Should I get a second opinion?

Most patients with Crohn's disease have a mild form of the disease that can easily be managed by a general gastroenterologist; however, some individuals have a more aggressive form of the disease. In particular, patients with extensive colitis and ongoing symptoms, despite the use of steroids or immunomodulators, are at increased risk for complications and might benefit from a second opinion.

Keep in mind that your healthcare provider wants you to get better and wants you to take an active role in your ongoing care. Don't be embarrassed to ask for a second opinion about treatment options, prognosis, or any aspect of their healthcare plan—it does not mean you don't trust your healthcare provider, it just means you want to learn more about your disease. You may be surprised to find that some insurance companies recommend or encourage patients to get second opinions. Some people choose to consult with a second healthcare provider when:

- They are considering surgery
- Their clinician prescribes a new medication
- They are not seeing an improvement in symptoms despite repeated visits to their healthcare provider
- They want to learn more about alternative treatments

There are multiple places to look when you are researching healthcare providers' credentials to find one to consult for a second opinion. Hospital Web sites list faculty members and their credentials, health insurance companies have lists of resources in your community, and even your healthcare provider can suggest other clinicians for you to see. Another resource is the CCFA, which provides a list of gastroenterologists with expertise in treating IBD. Hospitals may also list information about **clinical trials** that are testing new medications to treat CD. If you are interested, you might be eligible to participate. Information regarding current clinical trials can be found at http://www.clinicaltrials.gov.

Clinical trial

A controlled research study in which human volunteers test the safety and efficacy of new drugs or treatments.

Ask your clinician to send your medical records to the physician that will be providing a second opinion. If you will be bringing the records with you, it will be helpful to have notes from office visits, results from colonoscopies, and **pathology reports**. Also, for reference, plan to bring along original biopsy slides, X-rays, CT scans, and MRI scans. Ask the physician prior to your appointment, as they may be able to provide you with a list of items they would like you to bring.

Pathology reports

Results provided by a pathologist who describes the changes seen under the microscope on biopsied tissue.

20. Where can I get more information about Crohn's disease?

There are many resources available for people diagnosed with Crohn's disease. A list of useful organizations and their contact information is shown in **Table 4**. The Crohn's and Colitis Foundation of America (CCFA) has an information resource center that provides accurate and current disease-related information. The CCFA resource center is available to the public, healthcare professionals, patients, and their families. There are local CCFA chapters throughout the country that run educational programs as well as support groups. You can find a support group near you by searching the CCFA Web site or calling their toll-free number. You can also search for clinical trials in your area on the CCFA Web site, as well as at http://www.clinicaltrials.gov. Finally, you may wish to register with the CCFA to receive updates on research advances, new treatments, and other information that might be of use to you.

Be cautious about information that may not be based upon medically proven studies. It is important for patients to talk to their healthcare provider about food supplements or over-the-counter medications before starting them, to avoid adverse reactions or side effects.

Be cautious about information that may not be based upon medically proven studies.

Some of the drugs used to treat Crohn's disease can be very expensive, but resources to help pay for them are available. Pharmaceutical companies have web pages for their drugs that describe the **indications** (how the drugs are used to treat illnesses) and side effects, as well as information on how to apply for support to pay for them. Other resources about assistance for paying for specific medications include http://www.needymeds.org (215-625-9609) or http://www.rxassist.org/search/default.cfm (401-729-3284).

Indications

How a drug is used to treat a certain disease.

If you have insurance that requires costly co-pays, the Patient Advocate Foundation has a program to assist patients with ulcerative colitis (http://www.copays.org, or call 866-512-3861).

Table 4 Resources About Crohn's Disease

Name of Organization	Web site	Phone Number
American College of Gastroenterology	http://www.acg.gi.org	301-263-9000
American Gastroenterological Association	http://www.gastro.org	301-654-2055
Crohn's and Colitis Foundation of America	http://www.ccfa.org	800-932-2423
IBD Support Foundation	http://www.IBDSF.com	323-938-8090
The HealthCentral Network, Inc.	http://www.healthcentral.com/ibd/	703-302-1040
National Digestive Diseases Information	http://www2.niddk.nih.gov	800-891-5389
The Foundation for Clinical Research in IBD	http://www.MyIBD.org	
UC and Crohn's: A Site for Teens	http://www.ucandcrohns.org	
United Ostomy Associations of America	http://www.uoa.org	800-826-0826

5-ASAs: Aminosalicylates are medications used to treat the inflammation associated with inflammatory bowel disease; they come in oral and topical forms.

A

Abdomen/abdominal: Related to the area between the chest and the hips, consisting of the stomach, small intestine, large intestine, liver, gallbladder, pancreas, and spleen.

Abscess: An accumulation of pus.

Adhesion molecules: Proteins that help white blood cells stick to the lining of the intestines.

Anal fissure: A small tear in the anus that may cause itching, pain, or bleeding.

Anal ulcer: An ulcer within or just outside the anal canal.

Anastomosis/Anastomoses: A surgically-created connection of two normally separate organs.

Anemia: Decreased red blood cells.

Appendectomy: Operation to remove the appendix.

Appendicitis: Inflammation of the appendix, typically causing severe pain in the lower right side of the abdomen.

B

Backwash ileitis: Inflammation of the last few inches of the small intestine in ulcerative colitis patients with pancolitis.

Biologic agents: A group of therapeutic medications that include monoclonal antibodies.

Biopsy: A procedure in which a tiny piece of a body part, such as the colon, small intestine, or stomach, is removed for examination with a microscope.

Bloating: A fullness or swelling in the abdomen.

Bowel obstruction: A partial or complete blockage of the small or large intestine.

Bowel prep: Process used to clean the colon with enemas or a special drink that causes frequent bowel movements. It is used before surgery of the colon, a colonoscopy, or a barium enema X-ray.

C

Cecum: The first part of the large intestine.

Celiac disease: An immune reaction to gluten, a protein found in wheat, rye, and barley. The disease causes damage to the lining of the small intestine and prevents absorption of nutrients. Also called celiac sprue, gluten intolerance, and nontropical sprue.

Chromoendoscopy: A procedure in which dye is sprayed on the lining of the colon to make it easier to identify abnormalities during a colonoscopy.

Chronic: Lasting for a long time.

Clinical trial: A controlled research study in which human volunteers test the safety and efficacy of new drugs or treatments.

Clinician: A healthcare professional engaged in the care of patients.

Cognitive-behavioral therapy: A therapeutic approach that helps individuals take control of the way they respond to illness.

Colectomy: A surgical procedure to remove all or part of the colon.

Colon: Part of the large intestine extending from the cecum up to, but not including, the rectum. *See large intestine.*

Colonic CD: Crohn's disease isolated to the large intestine (colon and rectum).

Colonoscopy: A test to look into the rectum and colon that uses a long, flexible, narrow tube with a light and tiny camera on the end called a colonoscope.

Colorectal cancer: Cancer that starts in the colon (also called the large intestine) or the rectum (the end of the large intestine).

Colostomy: An operation that attaches the colon to an opening in the abdomen called a stoma. An ostomy pouch, attached to the stoma and worn outside the body, collects stool.

Corticosteroid: A type of medication given to reduce inflammation. Corticosteroids come in oral and topical forms.

Crohn's disease: A form of inflammatory bowel disease that causes inflammation in the gastrointestinal (GI) tract. It usually affects the lower small intestine (also called the ileum) or the colon, but it can also affect any part of the GI tract. Also called regional enteritis, granulomatous colitis, and ileitis. *See inflammatory bowel disease* and *granuloma.*

CT scan: An abbreviation for computed tomography, a technique of imaging body organs with detailed, cross-sectional views; it can be done with or without oral and intravenous contrast dye.

D

Diarrhea: Frequent, loose, and watery bowel movements. Causes include gastrointestinal infections, irritable bowel syndrome, inflammatory bowel disease, medicines, and malabsorption.

Diverticula: Plural for diverticulum, a small outpouching in the colon. These pouches are not painful and can become inflamed and lead to rectal bleeding.

Diverticulitis: A condition that occurs when small pouches in the colon, called diverticula, become inflamed.

Diverticulosis: A common condition in which tiny pouches of tissue, called diverticula, poke through weak areas of the colon.

Duodenum: The first part of the small intestine.

Dysplasia: A precancerous change in the lining of the gastrointestinal tract.

E

Elemental diet: A liquid diet of predigested nutrients used to treat patients with Crohn's disease.

Enema: The insertion of a liquid medication into the rectum and lower colon as a treatment.

Extraintestinal: Occurring outside of the intestines.

F

Fiber: A substance in foods that comes from plants. Fiber helps keep the stool soft so that it moves smoothly through the colon. Soluble fiber dissolves in water and is found in beans, fruit, and oat products. Insoluble fiber does not dissolve in water and is found in whole-grain products and vegetables.

Fibromyalgia: A chronic illness characterized by fatigue and widespread aching of muscles and soft tissues.

First-degree relative: Mother, father, sister, brother, son, or daughter.

Fissure: A tear in the lining of the anal canal.

Fistula/Fistulae: An abnormal passage between two organs, or between an organ and the outside of the body, caused when inflamed tissues come into contact and join together.

Fistulotomy: An operation performed by a surgeon to treat an anal fistula.

Flare: Worsening of symptoms of disease.

G

Gastroenterologist: A doctor who specializes in the diagnosis and treatment of digestive diseases.

Gastrointestinal (GI) tract: A large, muscular tube that extends from the mouth to the anus, where the movement of muscles, along with the release of hormones and enzymes, allows for the digestion of food. Also called the alimentary canal or digestive tract.

Genetic: Relating to biologic inheritance.

Gluten: A protein found in wheat, rye, and barley. In people with celiac disease, gluten damages the lining of the small intestine or causes sores on the skin. *See Celiac disease.*

Granuloma: Finding seen under the microscope in some patients with Crohn's disease.

Granulomatous colitis: Another name for Crohn's disease of the colon.

I

Ileitis: Inflammation of the small intestine. Several different disorders can cause inflammation of the small intestine.

Ileocolitis: Irritation of the lower part of the small intestine (ileum) and the beginning part of the colon.

Ileostomy: An operation that attaches the small intestine to an opening in the abdomen called a stoma. An ostomy pouch, attached to the stoma and worn outside the body, collects stool.

Ileum: The lower end of the small intestine.

Immune system: A complex and intertwined system of cells and genetics that controls the body's defense system against infection and other foreign organisms or substances.

Immunomodulators: A type of drug that is capable of modifying (decreasing or weakening) the effectiveness of the immune system.

Incontinence: Inability to control urination or defecation.

Indeterminate colitis: Inflammation of the colon that cannot be easily classified as either ulcerative colitis or Crohn's disease.

Indications: How a drug is used to treat a certain disease.

Infectious colitis: Inflammation of the colon caused by a bacteria, parasite, or virus.

Inflammation: Soreness, irritation, swelling.

Inflammatory bowel disease (IBD): A term for a variety of long-lasting disorders that cause inflammation in the gastrointestinal tract. The most common disorders are ulcerative colitis and Crohn's disease.

Intravenous (IV): Given into a vein.

Irritable bowel syndrome (IBS): A disorder associated with abdominal pain, bloating, and altered bowel habits. Also sometimes called spastic colon or mucous colitis.

Ischemic colitis: Inflammation of the colon caused by decreased blood flow. It may cause bloody diarrhea.

L

Lactose intolerance: Being unable to digest lactose, the sugar in milk.

Large intestine: Part of the intestine that includes the appendix, cecum, colon, and rectum. The large intestine absorbs water from the stool and changes it from a liquid to a solid. The large intestine is four feet long.

Left-sided colitis: Inflammation that extends from the rectum to the area above the sigmoid colon to the splenic flexure.

Lower bowel: Lower part of the colon that connects to the anus.

M

Metabolic panel: Blood tests that measure several components including sodium, potassium, chloride, bicarbonate, blood urea nitrogen (BUN), creatinine, liver tests, calcium, and glucose.

MRI scan: A magnetic resonance imaging (MRI) scan is a test that uses a magnetic field and pulses of radio wave energy to make pictures of organs and structures inside the body.

Mucosa: The lining of the gastrointestinal tract organs that absorbs nutrients and fluid, forms a barrier, and produces mucus.

Mucus: Clear to white liquid made by the intestines that coats and protects tissues in the gastrointestinal tract.

N

Nasogastric (NG) tube: A tube inserted through the nose, down the esophagus, and into the stomach.

Nocturnal: Occurring at night.

Nonsteroidal anti-inflammatory drugs (NSAIDs): A class of medications that can reduce pain, fever, and inflammation.

O

Ostomy: An operation that makes it possible for stool to leave the body through an opening made in the abdomen. An ostomy is necessary when part or all of the intestines are removed or blocked. Colostomy and ileostomy are types of ostomies.

Ova: The eggs of parasites.

P

pANCA: Anti-neutrophil cytoplasmic antibody blood test detected in autoimmune disorders.

Pancolitis: Inflammation that affects the entire inner lining of the colon.

Parasite: An infectious agent that lives in humans from which it obtains nutrition. Certain intestinal parasites can cause diarrhea and rectal bleeding.

pASCA: Anti-saccharomyces cerevisiae antibody blood test detected in autoimmune disorders.

Pathology reports: Results provided by a pathologist who describes the changes seen under the microscope on biopsied tissue.

Perforation: The breaking open of an organ.

Perianal: The area around the anus.

Polyp: An abnormal growth on the surface of the large or small intestine.

Prebiotics: Nondigestible food ingredients that are ingested by the normal bacteria occurring in the colon. They are believed to aid in digestion.

Primary sclerosing cholangitis (PSC): Irritation, scarring, and narrowing of the bile ducts inside and outside the liver. Bile builds up in the liver, damaging its cells and in some cases leading to cirrhosis. Many people with this condition also have inflammatory bowel disease.

Probiotics: Live beneficial bacteria found in food or diet supplements; they are believed to aid in digestion and may decrease gastrointestinal symptoms.

Proctitis: Inflammation of the rectum.

Prognosis: Prediction of the course of disease.

Psychotherapy: Treatment of emotional problems by a therapist using a variety of communication techniques.

R

Rectal bleeding: Bleeding that comes out through the anus.

Rectum: Lower end of the large intestine leading to the anus.

Regional enteritis: Another name for Crohn's disease.

Relapse: Disease symptoms that recur after being in remission.

Relaxation therapies: Techniques such as deep breathing or imagery that allow a person to relax and relieve anxiety.

Remission: Period of time when a disease does not cause symptoms.

Retention enema: Insertion of medicated fluids through the anus into the rectum and lower colon to help heal inflammation.

S

Sedation: Administration of medications during a test to reduce anxiety and discomfort.

Seton: A suture (material used during surgery to attach two structures to each other), made of thread or flexible wire, that is passed through a fistula to keep it open and prevent abscess formation.

Short bowel syndrome: Problems related to absorbing nutrients after removal of a long segment of the small intestine. Symptoms include diarrhea, weakness, and weight loss.

Sigmoid colon: Lower part of the colon that empties into the rectum.

Sigmoidoscopy: Looking into the sigmoid colon and rectum with a flexible tube called a sigmoidoscope.

Sitz bath: A special plastic tub that allows a person to sit in a few inches of warm water to help relieve the discomfort of hemorrhoids or anal fissures.

Small bowel X-ray: X-rays of the small intestine taken as barium liquid passes through the organ. Also called small bowel follow-through.

Small intestine: Organ where digestion and absorption occurs. It measures about 20 feet and includes the duodenum, jejunum, and ileum.

Stool: Solid waste that passes through the rectum as a bowel movement; it includes undigested food, bacteria, mucus, and dead cells. Also called feces.

Stricture: A narrowed area of intestine that develops due to chronic inflammation.

Stricturoplasty: An operation performed in patients with Crohn's disease to relieve obstruction of the small intestine without removal of the affected intestines.

Suppositories: A small plug of medication inserted in the rectum.

Suture: Material used during surgery to attach two structures.

T

Terminal ileitis: Another name for Crohn's disease.

Terminal ileum: Distal 1–2 feet of the ileum. It is attached to the colon by the ileocecal valve.

Toxic megacolon: Life-threatening complication usually from IBD that results in dilatation of the colon and possible perforation; may require emergency surgery to remove the colon.

Tumor necrosis factor (TNF): A type of protein that promotes inflammation in the body and gastrointestinal tract.

U

Ulcer: A sore on the skin's surface or on the stomach or intestinal lining.

Ulcerative colitis (UC): A disease that causes ulcers and irritation in the inner lining of the colon and rectum. *See inflammatory bowel disease.*

Upper GI series: X-rays of the esophagus, stomach, and duodenum. The patient swallows barium before X-rays are taken, as barium makes the organs show up on X-rays.

Urgency: The feeling of "needing to go" (either urine or stool).

Some glossary terms are courtesy of the National Digestive Diseases Information Clearinghouse, a service of the National Institute of Diabetes and Digestive and Kidney Diseases (NIDDK), National Institutes of Health (NIH): http://digestive.niddk.nih.gov/ddiseases/pubs/dictionary/.